Contents

Drug-Free Fixes:
Natural Solutions
for Pain Relief

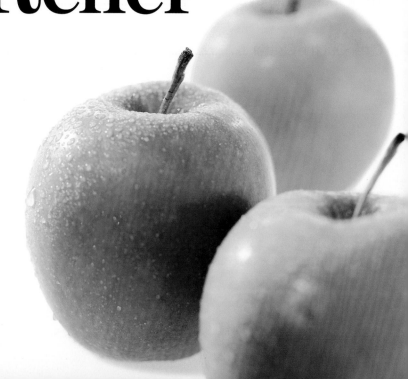

Your
Live Well,
Die Happy
Guides

Drug-Free Fixes:
Natural Solutions for Pain Relief

Think Yourself
Happy & Healthy

Clear Out the Clutter

The material here is designed to help you make informed decisions about your health. It is not intended as a substitute for any treatment that may have been prescribed by your doctor. If you suspect that you have a medical problem, please seek competent medical care.

Before you undertake a new health program or fitness regimen, we encourage you to discuss your plans with your health care professional, especially if you have not exercised for several years, are over 35, or are overweight.

Though self-healing is an important aspect of good health and general well-being, it is not meant to replace medical treatment or diagnosis. When illness strikes, we urge you to seek the best medical assistance that you can find.

Mention of specific companies, organizations, or authorities does not necessarily imply endorsement by the publisher, nor does it imply endorsement of the information by those companies, organizations, or authorities.

Project editor: Rachelle Laliberte
Project manager: Laura Mory
Copy editors: Leanne Sullivan, David Umla
Designer: Chris Rhoads
Photo editor: Jaime Livingood
Photography: Getty Images: front cover; Pure Ingredients: p. 4;
Mitch Mandel/Rodale: pp. 14–17; Augustus Butera: p. 20; Alamy: p. 33
Contributors: Stacey Colino, K. Aleisha Fetters, Hallie Levine Sklar, Jo Marchant, Jeannie Ralston, Tori Rodriguez, Karen Smith-Jannsen

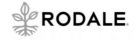

We inspire health, healing, happiness, and love in the world. Starting with you.

t's no wonder that, despite all the advances of modern medicine, home remedies have not just survived but thrived: They're inexpensive (even free!), convenient, and natural; and—most important—they work! In the pages that follow, you'll find drug-free solutions for common health problems and easy exercises to banish pain—plus discover the power of massage and other hands-on forms of healing.

Contents

Halt the Hurt— without Drugs

A compendium of cures to help banish common, annoying aches and persistent pains for good—no meds required

Back & Neck Pain

Back pain is the No. 2 reason that Americans see their doctors—second only to colds and flu. In fact, research shows that up to 90% of adults suffer from back pain at some time or other in their lives.

When it comes to your neck, seven vertebrae and 32 muscles do a good job of holding up your 10- to 12-pound head. Still, that's a heavy load resting on a relatively small structure, leaving your neck vulnerable to stresses that can result in pain.

The good news: There are many healing techniques you can use at home to ease the aches.

USE ICE, THEN HEAT Apply an ice pack wrapped in a thin cloth— such as a T-shirt—to the ache for 15 minutes at a time. After ice has reduced inflammation, use heat later on as a wonderful soother.

Try a heating pad, a heat wrap, or a hot bath or shower.

STAY ACTIVE Instead of getting caught up in your pain, try to resume your normal activities or do as much as you can do. It can be a little uncomfortable—you certainly don't want to create pain—but the sooner you can get back to your activities, the better you'll be.

EXERCISE, EVEN In a study at the Texas Tech University Health Sciences Center School of Nursing, researchers found that back pain patients who exercised returned to work more quickly than those who didn't. After a day or two of rest, begin light cardio training, such as walking, riding a stationary bicycle, or swimming. Aerobic activities can help blood flow to the area of pain and promote healing. They also strengthen muscles.

STRETCH OUT SPASMS Stretching will enhance the healing process. Lie on your back and gently bring your knees up to your chest. Once there, put a little pressure on your knees. Stretch, then relax. Repeat. You can also try gently stretching your body side to side and then forward and back.

PRESS ON Relieve muscle tension by applying moderate pressure to the area for 3 minutes. Don't press as hard as you can, but use your fingertips to exert steady, constant pressure on the affected point. At the end of 3 minutes, your pain may improve dramatically.

TURN TO HERBS Turmeric and ginger help reduce production of leukotrienes, substances that can trigger inflammation. Take 1 to 2 g of each herb a day in supplement form until your pain is relieved.

CREAM THE PAIN Capsaicin, the ingredient that gives cayenne its heat, can help ease muscle and joint aches. Studies show that it tamps down chemical messengers that transmit pain messages in the brain. Look for over-the-counter capsaicin ointments and creams, and follow package directions.

SPIKE YOUR JUICE Try this healthy addition: flax oil. Flaxseed contains alpha linolenic acid, a substance similar to the omega-3 fatty acids found in fish. Try 2 teaspoons a day. Make sure to refrigerate your flax oil—it spoils quickly.

WRAP UP When it's cold and damp outside, cover your neck well. The chilly weather can aggravate neck stiffness and pain.

POSITION YOURSELF RIGHT Sleeping on your stomach is bad for your back and neck. Instead, sleep in the fetal position—on your side with your knees pulled up toward your chest. Oftentimes, sleeping with a pillow between your knees can help prevent you from rolling onto your stomach. The pillow also stops your leg from sliding forward and rotating your hips, which puts added pressure on your back.

Each morning, when you're ready to get out of bed, slowly and carefully roll onto your side with your knees bent. Push yourself up with your arms or elbows into a seated position. Place your feet flat on the floor before you start to stand up. And move slowly, keeping your back as rigid as possible.

FIRM UP A firm mattress is important for spine alignment and support. If you don't have a firm mattress, try putting a ¾-inch piece of plywood between the mattress and the box spring to end the sagging problem.

SEE YOURSELF PAIN-FREE Close your eyes and imagine a pleasant scene. Think of yourself on a beach, for example, if that is a place that brings you peace. Bring as much detail to the image as possible until you can actually smell the ocean and feel the air. The more involved you are in the image, the quicker you will become distracted from the pain. This technique is especially helpful when pain wakes you in the middle of the night.

Earache

The stage is set for an ear infection when sinuses get clogged as a result of allergies or a head cold, or when the eustachian tubes become blocked by air pressure changes during an airplane descent. The best way to cure an ear infection is with antibiotics, although some infections clear up on their own, usually in a week to 10 days.

Other factors can cause earaches, too, including external otitis, or swimmer's ear, and odd things, such as tiny clippings from a haircut that fall into the ear canal and irritate your eardrum.

Whenever you experience ear discomfort, you need to see a doctor. But until you get there, here are some quick pain stoppers.

SIT UP Spending a few minutes sitting upright decreases swelling and makes your eustachian tubes start draining. Swallowing once you are sitting up also helps ease the pain. If it's possible, prop your head up slightly while you sleep to encourage better drainage.

GULP! Swallowing triggers the muscular action that helps your eustachian tubes open and drain. Open tubes mean less pain.

TAKE AN HERBAL APPROACH
Herbalists commonly recommend garlic and mullein oils for ear infections. Mullein is antimicrobial, and garlic works like an antibiotic. The oils will also migrate past the eardrum and help prevent further infections. You can buy garlic oil, mullein oil, or a combination of the two in most health food stores or drugstores. Apply 2 to 4 drops in the affected ear. Cover the ear with a little wad of cotton to keep the oil from running out. Apply more drops every 6 to 8 hours as needed. Use fresh cotton with each application. Caution: If you suspect that the eardrum may be ruptured or perhaps punctured, never drop fluids into your ear.

HEAT THINGS UP Warmth—a towel fresh from the dryer, a covered hot-water bottle, a heating pad set on low—can ease pain.

It may sound odd, but you can also try applying a warm plate to an aching ear. The heat feels really good as it radiates inward. Here's how to put the method to work: Microwave a small ceramic plate or saucer for a couple of seconds. It's ready when it's not too hot to the touch to take it out of the oven. Then place the plate gently cupped over the ear that hurts and hold it there.

CHEW GUM Most people know about this way to open their ears on a plane, but have you considered gum at other times? The muscular action of chewing may open the eustachian tubes.

YAWN Yawning also moves the muscles that open the eustachian tubes.

Gas

Uncomfortable—and sometimes embarrassing—gas is a common problem. Most cases can be traced back to diet. You may experience flatulence if your digestive system can't handle top offenders like lactose and certain carbohydrates. You probably know that beans are surefire flatus producers, but many more foods can also be highly flatulogenic.

Cabbage, broccoli, brussels sprouts, onions, cauliflower, whole wheat flour, radishes, bananas, apricots, and even pretzels can be at the bottom of gas problems.

As you make connections between episodes of gas and any food triggers, there are ways to ease the discomfort.

FIX IT WITH FENNEL Sugar-coated fennel seeds are served after meals in India just as Americans would have a mint. Look for them in gourmet shops and Asian food markets. Fennel is known as a carminative—an agent that can disperse gas from the intestinal tract. Try chewing ½ teaspoon of fennel seeds. The plain seeds (found in the spice aisle at the grocery store) can also be brewed as tea. Just cover 1 tablespoon with 1 cup of boiling water, strain, and sip.

TRY CHARCOAL Some studies have found that activated charcoal tablets are effective in eliminating excessive gas. Charcoal absorbs gases. Check with your doctor if you're taking any medication because charcoal can soak up medicine as well as gas.

SIP A SMOOTHIE Bitter herbs, like dandelion and chamomile, stimulate the production of enzymes that allow your body to digest food more fully and efficiently, so there's less for gas-producing bacteria to consume. Other foods that help are enzyme-rich pineapple and yogurt with live and active cultures. This smoothie recipe includes all of these digestive aids. In a blender, combine 1 cup pineapple chunks, 1 cup strawberries, ½ cup vanilla yogurt with live and active cultures, 1 teaspoon honey or maple syrup, ½ cup chamomile or dandelion root tea (cooled), and ½ cup ice cubes. Blend on high to the desired consistency.

Headache

It's a very rare—and lucky—person who has never experienced a headache. About 90% of all headaches are classified as tension headaches—they make you feel like there's a band wrapped around your head. Stress, lack of sleep, hunger, bad posture, and eyestrain are the most common causes of tension headaches.

An estimated 28 million Americans—nearly 10% of the population, and most of them women—suffer from migraines. Not "just a headache," a migraine is a complex condition that causes severe and often disabling head pain.

If your head starts throbbing, here are some expert recommendations to get rid of the pain and get back to your life.

WATER IT DOWN At the first twinge of pain, drink a cup or two of water. This tactic alleviated the headaches of 65% of sufferers within 30 minutes, reports a study in the journal *Headache*.

TAKE A NAP A lot of people sleep a headache off.

TRY A TENSION-ERASING TRICK Put a pencil between your teeth, but don't bite—you have to relax to do that. The relaxation—and distraction—could ease the headache.

ENLIST A BAND'S AID This old business of Grandmother tying a tight cloth around her head has some merit to it. Wearing a headband decreases blood flow to the scalp and lessens the throbbing and pounding of a migraine.

USE YOUR HANDS Two key pressure points for reducing pain with acupressure are the web between your forefinger and thumb (squeeze there until you feel pain) and under the bony bumps next to the ears on the back of the head (use each thumb to apply pressure there).

TRY VISUALIZATION Imagine the muscle fibers in your neck and head to be all scrunched up. Then begin to smooth them out in your mind.

GET A WHIFF OF THIS In one study, when people in the midst of a migraine attack sniffed test tubes containing green apple smell, the pain improved more than when they sniffed tubes that had no scent. Earlier studies found that the smell of green apples helps reduce anxiety.

ENJOY A LITTLE INTIMACY It might sound crazy, but 60% of migraine sufferers who had sex during an attack reported feeling better. The researchers speculate that feel-good hormones called endorphins may cause the pain to subside.

Heartburn

Eating too much food too fast is the most common cause of occasional heartburn. But it's not the only one. Certain foods, prescription medications, and stress can also trigger it.

Heartburn occurs when the acidic digestive juices normally found in the stomach flow backward—or reflux—up into the esophagus, making your chest feel as though it's on fire. To prevent that situation, eat smaller meals and limit fatty foods, citrus, onions, tomatoes, chocolate, and alcohol. Already feeling the heat? Try these tricks to extinguish it.

CHEW GUM Chewing gum can provide temporary relief of heartburn. It stimulates the flow of saliva, which neutralizes acid and helps push digestive juices back down where they belong. A small British study found that gum chewing doubles saliva production, and while it's not as efficient as taking an antacid, it is an all-natural remedy that's readily available in a pinch.

BET ON BANANA This naturally low-acid fruit is a great food to reach for if you're feeling the symptoms of heartburn. A banana forms a protective film that coats, protects, and soothes the irritated esophageal lining.

ENJOY ALMOND MILK You'll start your day off with fewer digestive issues if you blend an almond milk smoothie for breakfast. Almond milk is alkaline, so it helps neutralize acidic foods. To make a filling smoothie that tastes great, try blending together 1 cup each strawberries, spinach, and unsweetened almond milk and 1 frozen banana (for added creaminess).

GET HELP FROM GINGER This root is an excellent and age-old cure-all for many digestive ailments. Simply peel or grate an inch or so of ginger root and steep in boiling water to make a tea. You can also take it in capsule form.

TURN TO A GOOD ACID An oft-touted remedy for heartburn is 1 teaspoon of apple cider vinegar in a half glass of water sipped during a meal. It may sound bizarre to ingest an acid when you have an acid problem, but there are good acids and bad acids. For the best results, look for unfiltered apple cider vinegar that contains the sediment.

STAY (SORT OF) UPRIGHT If you lie down flat, you'll have gravity working against your body's efforts to keep the acid down. To help, elevate the head of your bed 4 to 6 inches. Put blocks under the legs of the bed or slip a wedge under the mattress at the head of the bed. (Extra pillows, however, don't always do the trick.)

LIE ON YOUR LEFT The esophagus enters the stomach on your right side. Sleeping on your left side prevents any remaining food in your stomach from pressing on the opening to the esophagus, which could lead to reflux.

Joint Pain

When joint pain flares up, you want relief—fast. If you're looking to add a drug-free remedy to your arsenal, ice and heat are great, but they're not your only options.

TAKE TO THE WATER A review in the journal *Physical Therapy* found that exercising in water reduces pain and improves physical functioning in people with osteoarthritis of the lower limbs. Meanwhile, a study from the Netherlands found that a 45-minute aquatic circuit training session helped relieve the pain of knee osteoarthritis.

WORK OUT ALL OUT It's counterintuitive, but hard workouts can also be salve for achy joints. When women with rheumatoid or osteoarthritis sweated through 30 minutes of indoor cycling intervals twice a week, they slashed indicators of pain-causing inflammation in their blood by an average of nearly 40% after 10 weeks, according to a study in the *European Journal of Applied Physiology*. They also lost weight, dropped body fat, and increased their stamina without any negative side effects.

SPICE THINGS UP Capsaicin, a substance responsible for the heat in hot peppers, is used in topical pain relievers. A study from Case Western Reserve University found that 80% of people with rheumatoid or osteoarthritis had less pain after applying capsaicin cream four times a day for 2 weeks.

CONSIDER SUPPLEMENTS Glucosamine and chondroitin sulfate (both found in human cartilage) are popular for treating the pain and swelling associated with osteoarthritis. Studies on their effectiveness have been mixed, but a research review determined that this combo significantly reduces pain and improves functioning in people with osteoarthritis of the knee.

GO FISH It's no secret that omega-3 fatty acids, including fish oil supplements, have anti-inflammatory properties. A study from Thailand found that when people with osteoarthritis of the knee took 1,000 mg of fish oil supplements (a combination of EPA, or eicosapentaenoic acid, and DHA, or docosahexaenoic acid) once a day for 8 weeks, their pain decreased and their functioning improved significantly.

Sinusitis

Pressure and pain around the face, teeth, or eyes, and often a headache and a thick green or yellow nasal discharge, are the hallmarks of acute sinusitis. You may run a fever as well. Acute sinusitis is usually caused by viruses or bacteria and can last a month or longer. Less common than acute sinusitis, chronic sinusitis is caused by allergies or other conditions and typically lasts longer than 8 weeks.

Doctors generally prescribe antibiotics to clear an infection if it's bacterial. However, they often suggest you wait it out for a week, because about three-quarters of sinus infections will improve without prescription medications. In the meantime, you can take a number of steps to feel better.

GET STEAMED UP Put a few drops of eucalyptus oil on the floor of a hot, running shower. Inhale the steam. The humidity will help keep the mucus flowing and your sinuses drained. This could be slippery, so be careful getting into and out of the shower.

BATHE YOUR NOSTRILS To flush out stale nasal secretions, try using saline nasal sprays or drops. Or make your own solution by mixing 1 teaspoon of table salt and a pinch of baking soda into 2 cups of warm water. Pour the liquid into a squirt bottle or medicine dropper, tilt your head back, close one nostril with your thumb, and squirt the solution into the open nostril while sniffing. Then blow that nostril gently. Repeat on the other side. You can also use a mister to spray the solution into your nostrils, but keep your head in an upright position.

HEAD TO THE KITCHEN Eating foods that make your eyes water or nose run can help clear your sinuses. Try:

- **Garlic.** This herb contains the same chemical found in a drug that makes mucus less sticky.

- **Horseradish.** This pungent root contains a chemical similar to one found in decongestants. The bottled variety works just fine.

- **Hot peppers.** Hot peppers, like cayenne chiles, contain capsaicin, a substance that can stimulate the nerve fibers and may act as a natural nasal decongestant. Or use ground red pepper (cayenne) or other ground chile powders in cooking.

APPLY PRESSURE Rubbing your sore sinuses brings a fresh blood supply to the area for soothing relief. Press your thumbs firmly on both sides of your nose and hold for 15 to 30 seconds. Repeat.

PT-Approved Pain-Fighting Moves

Seven simple strengtheners to knock out pain

Got a nagging ache? Recovering from a sprain? The person you most want to talk to is a physical therapist: They improve bodies for a living. They know an important secret: strength training. Research suggests that not only is strength training the best way to knock out pain, but like a magic pill it can also prevent pain in the first place. "People often only think of exercise as a way of building muscle, until they get hurt," says Alonzo Wilson, founder of fitness studio Tone House New York and a former pro athlete. "Once you go to physical therapy, you find out that exercise is also a way to prevent and recover from injury."

You'll need a chair, a small towel, a heavy household object (such as a bag of flour or a hefty book), and a yoga mat to do these trainer-approved pain-pill moves.

1. For Feet: Towel Curls

WORKS: PLANTAR FLEXORS

Sit on a chair with your bare feet flat on the ground and a small towel beneath your feet, as shown. Using your toes, pinch the towel and pull it toward you, moving it just a few inches. Release the towel and relax your foot. You can make this move tougher by putting a weight on the edge of the towel. Do 3 sets of 8 to 10 reps with each foot.

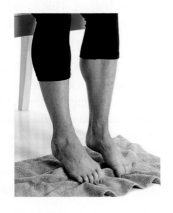

2. For Neck: Neck Rolls

WORKS: CERVICAL SPINE, TRAPEZIUS

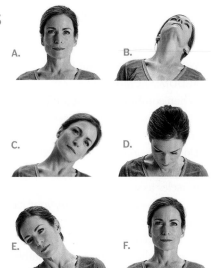

Stand with good posture, shoulders relaxed, as shown. Slowly tilt your head to the left, then roll it forward until you're looking down in front of you. Continue to rotate your head around until you arrive back at the starting position. That's 1 rep. (You can increase resistance by placing your hands lightly on the back of your head.) Do 3 sets of 8 to 10 reps.

3. For Knees: Chair Squats

WORKS: QUADRICEPS, HAMSTRINGS, GLUTEUS MAXIMUS, OBLIQUES, ABDOMINAL MUSCLES

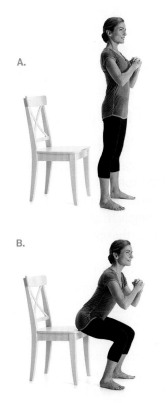

Chair squats help prevent and even ease knee pain by strengthening the leg muscles around the knees. "If those muscles are weak, your knees will be unstable," says Krista Stryker, a San Francisco–based personal trainer and creator of the 12-Minute Athlete HIIT program and app.

Stand in front of a chair with your feet about hip-width apart and hands clasped in front of you, as shown. Bend at the knees and slowly lower your body until you're sitting on the front part of the chair; at the same time, bend your arms and bring your fists to your chest. Keeping your weight on your heels, stand back up. That's 1 rep. (To increase the difficulty, use a lower chair or decrease your speed.) Do 3 sets of 8 to 10 reps.

4. For Shoulders:
Shoulder Presses

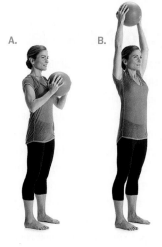

A.　　　　B.

**WORKS: DELTOIDS, TRICEPS,
ABDOMINAL MUSCLES**

When combined with stability exercises like planks, shoulder presses are one of the best ways to protect your shoulders, says Stryker. Doing the presses standing rather than sitting forces you to recruit your abdominal muscles as well, she says.

Stand with good posture, your feet about hip-width apart, and hold any sort of heavy household object—a big book, a bag of flour, a weighted backpack—at your chest, as shown. The more unstable the weight is, the more it will work your muscles. (You can also use a long resistance band by stepping on the center and holding the ends at your chest.) Tighten your core and keep your back straight as you press your arms straight above your head until your elbows are almost locked, lifting your shoulders up as far as possible at the top of the movement. Hold for 1 to 2 seconds, then slowly lower the object back down. Do 3 sets of 12 to 15 reps.

5. For Upper Back:
Lying Upper-Back Squeeze

**WORKS: TRAPEZIUS, RHOMBOIDS,
ERECTOR SPINAE**

A.

This simple movement strengthens smaller muscles in the upper back and shoulders.

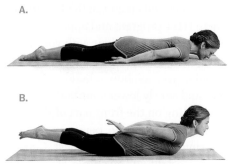

B.

Lie on your stomach with your arms at your sides, as shown. Raise your chest and shoulders off the floor. With your palms up, bring your hands together behind your back until your thumbs touch (or almost touch), squeeze your shoulder blades together. Return to the starting position; that's 1 rep. Do 3 sets of 12 to 15 reps.

6. For Hips: Hip Bridges

WORKS: HIPS, GLUTES, ABS

This move comes courtesy of Hollywood celebrity trainer Teddy Bass. To address imbalances in your hips, he says, you need to either strengthen weak muscles or stretch tight muscles—and this move does both.

Lie on your back with your feet flat on the floor, hip-width apart. Flatten your lower back, then exhale and raise your hips toward the ceiling with the help of your abs. Hold for 2 or 3 seconds, squeezing through your glutes, then inhale and lower your hips back to the floor. (You can increase the challenge by lifting one leg while your hips are in the raised position.) Do 2 or 3 sets of 8 to 10 reps.

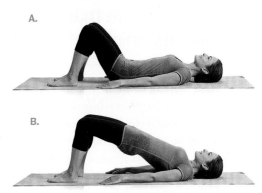

7. For Lower Back: Cow/Cat Pose

WORKS: LOWER SPINE, HIPS, BACK, CORE

Start on all fours with your hands directly under your shoulders and knees under your hips. As you inhale, drop your belly toward the floor, lift your rear and chest upward, and raise your head and gaze forward (A). As you exhale, round your spine upward like a stretching cat while you let your head hang toward the floor (B); that's 1 rep. Do 8 to 10 reps.

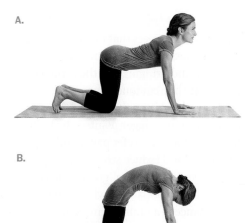

The Right Touch for Healing

Massage is more than a soothing retreat. Discover its unique effects for pain relief.

A rubdown can be more than a luxury, whether you're in the hands of a family member who's massaging your neck while you sit in the living room recliner or a masseuse who's kneading your sore muscles with scented aromatherapy oils in the hush of a beautiful spa. This form of therapy can really work against many types of pain.

Massage brings welcome relief from headaches if neck muscles are tight, eases backaches, and even soothes cancer pain. It can help you sleep better so that coping with pain and getting on with your life are easier. The unique, prolonged human contact also brings a sense of well-being and calm that's hard to find when you spend your days (and nights) fending off pain, restoring a sense of peace so that pain is no longer the center of your life.

Power against Pain

Researchers suspect that in addition to relaxing stiff muscles, boosting circulation, reducing swelling, and bringing you the comfort of compassionate human touch, massage erases pain on deeper levels, too. It can relieve pressure on nerves, turn off trigger points—the highly sensitive areas that may refer pain to other parts of the body—and reduce stress. There's evidence it raises levels of the feel-good brain chemicals serotonin and dopamine while it lowers levels of substance P, a brain chemical linked with higher pain intensity in people with lower-back pain, fibromyalgia, and arthritis. Massage also promotes deeper sleep.

Headache Halter

Rubbing your temples with mint oil can melt the immediate pain of a tension headache. Regular massage can do far more, cutting in half the number of headaches suffered by chronic head pain sufferers in one study published in the *American Journal of Public Health*.

According to research, massage may help with back and shoulder pain, cancer pain, and tension headaches and may also ease fibromyalgia and neck pain. And by helping you relax, it eases the stress that can make any type of chronic pain feel even worse.

Making the Most of Massage

Massage works best in combination with other chronic pain treatments, including medications, acupuncture, exercise, and mind-body therapies. You probably won't be able to trade in your pain-relieving drugs for an hour on a comfy massage table, but combining this hands-on therapy with your current treatment regimen may help ease pain more than drugs alone can. And it might even allow you to reduce your dose.

There are many types of massage out there. What's best for pain? In one study of people with cancer pain, four types of rubdowns—classic deep-tissue massage; the long, gliding strokes of Swedish massage; light-touch massage; and simple foot rubs—all helped people feel better. Another type, myofascial release, targets tight spots in the fascia—a stringy, spongy tissue that connects muscles, skin, and organs throughout your body—to ease muscle-, joint-, and nerve-related pain conditions, such as back pain, carpal tunnel syndrome, fibromyalgia, shoulder problems, headaches, and foot pain.

It's important to work with a licensed and/or certified massage therapist with experience and training in chronic pain. Talk with your doctor about types of massage that are (or are not) right for you and any areas of your body the therapist should skip.

More Hands-On Healers

Hot/cold therapy: Heat therapy—with heat patches, a warm bath or shower, or a warm, moist towel—expands blood vessels, boosts circulation, and relaxes tense muscles. In contrast, cold therapy—with a cold pack, a sealed bag of ice cubes, or a bag of frozen vegetables wrapped in a towel—can numb deep muscle pain and prevent or soothe inflammation. Some people find alternating is best; others prefer one over the other.

The MELT Method: Short for *myofascial energetic lengthening technique*, this cross between self-massage and exercise uses rubber balls and foam rollers to relieve tight areas in your fascia.

Reiki: In this ancient Japanese healing art, a practitioner works to free energy flow by lightly touching, tapping, or moving his arms above your body and focusing on seven key areas called chakras.

Think
Yourself
Happy
&Healthy

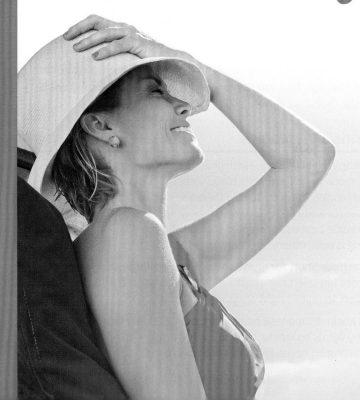

You've likely heard a lot about mindfulness, but what exactly is it? It's a mental state in which you focus on awareness and the present moment—a simple notion that takes a lot of practice. But it's worth the effort. When you live more mindfully, you can live life more fully. Read on to find out how.

Contents

Grounded, Happy, and Healthy

Mindfulness changes the brain and body for the better.

Most of us spend a large proportion of our waking hours (47%, according to one study) engaged in what psychologists call mind wandering. We're running on autopilot while daydreaming or caught up in thoughts about the past or future, whether it's replaying an argument or planning what to make for dinner.

Mindfulness is essentially the opposite: consciously turning our attention to whatever we're doing, thinking, or feeling at a particular moment. It's important to do this neutrally, without judgment, noticing thoughts or sensations with detached interest before letting them go.

You're not alone if you find mindfulness difficult. In one study, 67% of men and 25% of women chose to administer painful electric shocks to themselves rather than try to cope with being left alone with their thoughts. Masters of mindfulness suggest that if we practice regularly, we gain more control over our conscious minds, which in turn reduces our stress.

Research is finally catching up with these long-held beliefs—and revealing even more benefits. One way to study the effects is by scanning and examining people's brains while they meditate. In some of the earliest research of this type, conducted on Buddhist monks who had spent tens of thousands of hours meditating, scientists observed high levels of activity in brain areas that control focus and positive emotions. It wasn't clear whether such effects were attainable for the rest of us, however, so Sara Lazar, a Harvard University neuroscientist, pioneered a different approach.

In two studies, she asked volunteers with little or no experience with meditation to take an 8-week mindfulness meditation course. She and her coauthors surprised the scientific community by showing that mindfulness didn't just alter the volunteers' brain activity to become more monklike while they meditated. It also changed the physical structure of their brains.

Together with other studies carried out since, the results suggest that mindfulness training can help repair damage done by stress, reshaping the brain in a way that makes us better able to regulate our emotions and more resilient to stress in the future.

Mounting evidence also shows that mindfulness training can ease physical symptoms such as pain and fatigue. In one of the largest mindfulness studies ever conducted, for example, 61% of patients with chronic pain who received mindfulness training said their pain improved and the improvements lasted at least a year.

These findings raise an intriguing possibility. Stress creates a cascade of physiological changes (known as the fight-or-flight response) that trigger inflammation, the body's first line of defense against infection and injury. Heightened inflammation can be lifesaving in an emergency—but inflammation caused by chronic stress makes wounds heal more slowly, worsens autoimmune diseases, and increases susceptibility to infection. Chronic inflammation is also linked to some cancers and faster cell aging.

So can stress-busting mindfulness stop us from becoming ill in the first place? The research in this area is more preliminary, but there is some tantalizing evidence to support the idea. A trial of 154 people found that, compared with a control group, volunteers who practiced mindfulness had fewer colds, and when they did get sick, their symptoms were less severe and didn't last as long. Several studies have also found that mindfulness training reduces markers of inflammation in the blood and boosts activity of an enzyme called telomerase, which slows cell aging.

We don't have the full picture yet, and we know that mindfulness doesn't appeal to everyone. But so far it looks like mindfulness does help to reverse not just the psychological consequences of stress but the physical ones, too.

Which leaves one last question: How much mindfulness meditation do we need to do? Some studies have seen small, brief effects on mood and pain after as little as 5 to 10 minutes per day for 3 or 4 days. The effects of lengthier mindfulness courses seem to be more significant and longer lasting. Rather than seeing mindfulness as a miracle cure, then, think of it as a lifestyle change like exercise or healthy eating: The more you do, the greater the impact, and the benefits last as long as you keep practicing.

Mindful in a Moment

For a quick mindfulness meditation, close your eyes for 60 seconds and pay attention to your breathing, experiencing the sensation of air moving in and out of your nose. If you notice your mind straying, return your focus to your breath.

Live in the Now— Here's How

The secret to great health might lie in a surprising place—the present.

Practicing more mindfulness could mean major health benefits: You can reduce stress, boost your brain, and power up your body. No wonder so many people are turning to it to, for example, relieve anxiety, improve sleep, and help weight loss.

"Mindfulness has gone from a niche practice to something embraced by tens—if not hundreds—of millions of people," says Danny Penman, PhD, coauthor of *Mindfulness: An Eight-Week Plan for Finding Peace in a Frantic World*. And per researchers, it works—with no negative side effects.

Presence of Mind

It's a concept that is simultaneously super simple and difficult to grasp. "Mindfulness is a full awareness of precisely what is happening in the present," says Penman. Think of it like this: Most of us spend a lot of time either mulling over the past (*"If only I'd kept my mouth shut ..."*) or worrying about the future (*"Will I ever finish this assignment?"*). Mindfulness involves stilling that chatter and focusing on the here and now, says psychologist Susan Albers, PsyD, a mindfulness expert at the Cleveland Clinic. "It is concentrating on what's happening in the moment, without dwelling, judging, or trying to change anything."

In other words, no overthinking or overanalyzing—or the opposite, banishing all thoughts. Unlike many forms of meditation, which involve totally clearing your mind, mindfulness means letting your thoughts come and go without rushing to figure out what they mean.

If that sounds a little too Zen, keep in mind that you can't be mindful all the time. There is, however, a cumulative and lasting effect. "Mindfulness is both a process and an outcome," says Mirabai Bush, of the Center for Contemplative Mind in Society. "The day-to-day practice leads to a general state of heightened awareness." It also leads to some awesome health boons.

Start Your Practice

Best of all: Mindfulness is free. Caveat: It takes loads of practice. But before the idea of more work makes you turn away, consider that you can try it anytime, anyplace, in almost any situation. And once you get the hang of it, you'll automatically be more mindful, without much effort.

To start, try to set aside 10 to 20 minutes a day. Remember that "you'll never be able to spend tons of time in a state of mindfulness; the human mind is designed to wander, and that's OK," says Penman. So don't give yourself a mental spanking if you break your concentration. Keep at it with these step-by-step tips.

JUST BREATHE The very thing that makes mindfulness so accessible—you can do it anywhere—is also what can make it seem confusing. The simplest place to begin is with your breath, says Diana Winston, director of mindfulness education at UCLA's Mindful Awareness Research Center. Sit or stand in a comfortable, quiet place and breathe naturally. No need to count inhalations and exhalations; just relax, focusing on the sensations in your stomach, chest, or nostrils. If your mind wanders, gently bring your attention back to your breath.

USE WHAT YOU'VE GOT Next, try bringing that "here and now" awareness to everyday activities. For example, notice the warmth of the water and movement of your hands while washing the dishes; focus on how the bristles feel on your gums while brushing your teeth; observe the leaves, grass, and smells around you on a nature walk.

FIND YOUR CENTER Start employing that focus in ordinary real-life situations. Take your mental temperature throughout the day. If you notice you are, for example, stressed about an upcoming work meeting, spend a few minutes in mindful breathing. Don't try to push your anxious thoughts away; rather, try watching your mind in action. Acknowledge your stress and where it's stemming from. This helps dissolve negativity, says Penman.

GET READY FOR PRIME TIME You can try mindfulness in higher-stakes scenarios, such as a confrontation with a friend. Practice mindful breathing beforehand, and then, even in the thick of conversation, stay aware of your breath, body, and emotions. Remain in the moment rather than jumping ahead to how you'll respond or fend off a verbal bruising. This will help you be a better listener and avoid saying anything you'll later regret.

KNOW HOW TO STOP If at any point you get frustrated—hey, it happens, even to the pros—fall back on the STOP method: *Stop, Take a breath, Observe* what's happening inside and around you at that moment, then *Proceed* with whatever you're doing. Eventually, your default emotional setting will be calmer—and your body and mind will thank you.

Wander Mindfully in the Woods

Research shows that spending quality time with foliage can slay stress, nix negative thoughts, and fortify the immune system.

iddy is not a word that brings John Muir immediately to mind. Nature is supposed to be stately, serene, serious. But go take a walk and observe what really happens. You may skip. You may trip, then laugh at yourself. You may make crazy faces when you hear a birdcall.

Such antics are not the only human behaviors you'll observe in nature. But being high on nature—in the throes of what's sometimes called (too cutely) outdoorphins and vitamin G (for *green*)—essentially means being in a supreme comfort zone, say scientists, a place of freedom where it's OK to act as if we've been drinking beverages made from fermented plants. We evolved to enjoy places rich in natural resources because they represented a good turn of events. Richard Ryan, PhD, a professor of psychology at the University of Rochester, has researched how being outdoors can even make us nicer. "In nature," he says, "we feel more in touch with who we really are and what we want to do."

Who you are, apparently, is someone pretty spectacular, someone more energized and generous (studies have found both), unjangled (a study showed that long walks through forests over 2 days lowered stress-hormone levels, pulse rate, and blood pressure), vital (after just 20 minutes a day in nature, according to one of Ryan's studies), and ecstatic (neuroscientists say viewing natural settings increases interactions in the brain's pleasure receptors). And likely less blue: The University of Essex in the UK found that 30 minutes of walking in a green scene reduced depression in 71% of participants.

The reason being outdoors performs like a drug may be, astonishingly, because you are floating in quasi-pharmaceuticals. This is the gist of research into the microbes of nature. A Japanese researcher has zeroed in on airborne antifungal and antibacterial compounds called phytoncides. Inhaling these seems to boost a type of white blood cell that attacks tumors and viruses. (People living in heavily forested areas of Japan have lower rates of mortality from several types of cancer.) His finding has contributed to a national pastime known as forest bathing: Millions of Japanese walk along 48 Forest Therapy trails annually for relief from what ails them in the country's notoriously crowded cities. Researchers have also flagged another inhaled substance, the harmless soil microbe *M. vaccae*, which works as a natural Zoloft and stimulates the release of cytokines, which can in turn lead to the production of serotonin in the mood-regulating area of the brain.

It's not hard to pull off such happy interventions, according to scientists. Getting out into any park is fine, especially if you spend time under trees, rather than in open fields, for maximum phytoncide intake. And slow down—preferably without being plugged into a smartphone—so that all five senses can get their share (it's OK to run your fingers through soil). "The effects are enhanced if you're paying close attention to nature, immersing yourself," says Ryan.

Even in the city, you can grow phytoncide-emitting houseplants or get a bliss bump just from looking at photos of gorgeous scenery—which may explain why, say, a dentist's office might have a waterfall poster on the ceiling. More good news for the building-bound: The forest-bathing research team found that aromatherapy, such as whiffing cypress essential oil, can also deliver phytoncides for a little hit of happiness.

Get Nurtured in Nature

Walking or sitting in nature, aka *Shinrin-yoku*, started in Japan but is spreading like (dare we say it) wildfire to US wellness spas. Here's why you shouldn't wait for a trip to Sedona to try it.

- **It's great for your heart.** A few hours in nature lowers blood pressure—and the stress hormones cortisol and adrenaline.

- **It soothes your brain.** Being in greenery decreased anxiety, depression, anger, and fatigue for adults in one study. Other research shows that kids with ADHD who spend time in natural outdoor environments have a reduction in symptoms.

- **It speeds recovery.** People in the hospital given green views after surgery had shorter stays, took fewer painkillers, and had fewer complications than those who stared out at a cement wall.

- **It beefs up immunity.** When you inhale fresh forest air, you breathe in phytoncides, plant chemicals that have antibacterial and antifungal qualities and increase the immune system's disease-fighting natural killer cells.

Approach the Day Thoughtfully

Is your brain a beehive of activity? This hour-by-hour guide will help you find peace in your frantic life so you can recapture the joy.

Are you frequently multitasking, even though research shows that our minds are not meant to? (One study finds that multitasking can even temporarily lower your IQ as much as if you'd lost a night's sleep.) If you're still struggling to cram everything you can into a 24-hour cycle, stop. Calm down, take a deep breath, and let health and wellness experts offer you the ideal, sometimes surprising, times to do almost anything.

Make the Most of Morning

7 AM: GET INTIMATE Instead of reaching for the snooze button, reach for your partner. Men's and women's testosterone levels (which play a big role in arousal) are at their peak first thing in the morning and lowest around bedtime, when most people have sex.

7:30 AM: WEIGH IN Jump on the scale at the same time once or twice a week, advises Lisa Young, PhD, RD, an adjunct professor of nutrition and food studies at New York University. To stay upbeat, nix daily checks—temporary bumps can discourage weight loss efforts.

7:35 AM: BREAK A SWEAT Rather than wait for a weekend treadmill session, take a brisk pre-breakfast walk instead. You'll burn more fat because you haven't yet consumed any carbs, so the body can't turn to them first for energy. An early workout can also help you stick to your fitness goals. "You're less likely to skip out on exercise if you do it in the morning," says G. Ryan Shelton, MD, medical director of internal medicine at Mecklenburg Medical Group SouthPark in Charlotte, NC. Plus, it adds mental focus and energy to the start of your day. If you can get outside, even better. Early-morning sun helps your body naturally reset to a healthier sleep/wake cycle. (Regular indoor lights don't have the same effect.)

8 AM: EAT BREAKFAST Time your morning meal to within an hour or two of getting up. "Waiting too long to eat breakfast can cause your blood sugar to dip," Young says, adding that you'll feel famished later. If you have a high-protein breakfast, you'll eat less later in the day.

9 AM: SEE A DOCTOR You can avoid a long wait if you make an early appointment, before your doctor encounters distractions or other appointments that run long, says Shelton. Try to get your flu shot early, too. University of Birmingham researchers found that people who were vaccinated between 9 and 11 AM had a higher antibody response, which implies they may gain more protection than those who receive vaccinations in the afternoon.

10 AM: POUR YOUR FIRST COFFEE Your usual habit of reaching for the java as you're turning off your alarm is unwise, says sleep specialist and clinical psychologist Michael J. Breus, PhD, author of the book *The Power of When*. "On first waking, you have high levels of the stress hormone cortisol,

which makes you feel more awake and alert. If you add caffeine, all you're doing is making yourself feel jittery," he says.

11 AM: DIVE IN TO A TASK Tackle a big project, do your taxes, finish your novel, or just work on a crossword puzzle. You're at your sharpest mentally by midmorning, when your grogginess is gone (and by now you're fully caffeinated, since coffee's effects kick in after about 10 minutes and last 4 to 6 hours). Productivity is also high because the activity is still relatively new—the longer we work at something, the less efficient we become. If you tackle tough work now, Breus says, you'll get it done in record time.

Ace Your Afternoon

12 PM: EAT LUNCH Aim to eat your midday meal about 4 hours after having breakfast, Young says. And if you can, enjoy another walk for 10 to 15 minutes before you take a bite. This will tamp down your appetite so you'll make healthier choices at lunch as well as avoid your coworker's candy bowl later on, adds Breus.

1 PM: FILL YOUR FRIDGE According to a Cornell University study published in *JAMA Internal Medicine*, hungry shoppers fill their carts with more calories. Food shopping in the hours post-lunch and presnack—or between 1 and 4 PM—resulted in a lower calorie total for groceries than shopping closer to dinnertime. A bonus in the early afternoon, says Young, is fresher produce, because employees restock shelves with new shipments in the late morning.

2 PM: TAKE A NAP Now is the time to steal some shut-eye. You can reinvigorate yourself with 15 minutes of rest, according to Breus. Stick to a short snooze so you don't enter deep sleep; otherwise, you can end up feeling groggier than when you started.

3 PM: MAKE A BIG DECISION Aim extra brainpower at your biggest problem in midafternoon, when emotion, hunger, and fatigue have the least chance of clouding your judgment. "You want to have some oomph in you but not be overwhelmed by stress," says psychologist Elizabeth Lombardo, PhD. While you're deciding, you may want to skip the trip to the ladies' room. In a study published in the journal *Psychological Science*, people tasked with finding solutions on a full bladder tended to make better decisions, thanks to what the researchers called "increased impulse control in the behavioral domain."

4 PM: ATTACK A SNACK Midafternoon nibblers pick healthier bites, according to a University of Illinois at Chicago study published in the *Journal of the American Dietetic Association.* The researchers found that afternoon snackers ate more fiber, fruit, and veggies than morning snackers did and also lost more weight. Young's advice: Grab a snack more than 2 hours after you ate your last meal to help keep you satisfied during the hours between lunch and dinner.

Ensure a Great Evening

7 PM: EAT DINNER Your last meal of the day should also be the smallest—and, best-case scenario, finished before 8 PM. Eating within 3 hours of bedtime can lead to digestive trouble and disrupted sleep, Young says.

8 PM: POST ON SOCIAL MEDIA This is prime time for social networking, when posts get the most likes, shares, and comments. It's also a healthy time to post. You're staring at the screen far enough from bedtime that the screen time won't disturb your sleep cycle—or your mood. The more time you spend browsing social media sites, the more likely you are to get depressed, according to new research. "Social media posts aren't what you want to put into your mind right before you go to sleep," Lombardo says.

9 PM: TUNE IN TO THE TUBE When you push back your bedtime to squeeze in "just one more episode," it confuses your brain, which is accustomed to entering sleep mode at a particular time. If you must catch up on a show, finish your screen session—which includes your computer and your phone—by 10 PM to ensure restful sleep.

10 PM: TAKE A BATH Now that you've powered down your devices, a late-evening bath is a great way to power yourself down. Core body temperature naturally drops at night, signaling the brain that sleep is on the way. A warm bath artificially raises body temperature; then, when you get out of the tub, the exaggerated cooldown is a clear sign that it's time for bed.

10:30 PM: MEDITATE Continue your calming ritual with a short meditation to lower your blood pressure, heart rate, and cortisol level, which further prepares you to fall asleep.

11 PM: CALL IT A NIGHT While sleep needs vary from person to person, between 7 and 9 hours is considered optimal for healthy adults, according to the National Sleep Foundation. Experts advise calculating your bedtime in 90-minute sleep cycles. Ideally, you'd complete at least four cycles each night, though five is even better.

11:20 PM: GET OUT OF BED If you're wide awake 20 minutes or more after tucking in, get up. Resist the urge to peek at a screen, which will further interrupt your sleep. Calm yourself by reading, meditating, or doing breathing exercises. Keep the lights dim. After 10 to 15 minutes, head back to bed and try again. Sweet dreams, and please don't try to fall asleep by counting the things on your to-do list or you'll undo the equilibrium you've gained by following this guide to good timing.

Clear Out the Clutter

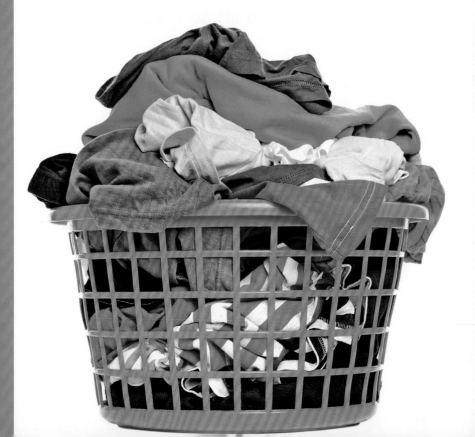

t's safe to say that, if you live in your home, you live with clutter. Those design-magazine photos of immaculate rooms with empty shelves and one perfectly placed *objet d'art* on the coffee table are essentially sets, unlived in and unloved. Clutter is simply part of the human condition. But you're stuck with the messy, stacked-up status quo. You can pare down the piles (and maybe even yourself!), thanks to the following tips and tricks from pros who know how to sift, sort, and say "so long" to the stuff.

Contents

Enough with the Stuff!

Can you love your things too much? Absolutely! Use these tips to break free from the emotional pull possessions have over you.

Being clingy isn't just deadly in relationships—it's also bad news when it comes to your possessions. The megahit TV series *Hoarders* has led to a weird fascination with the problem of having way too much stuff, but you don't have to be a full-blown hoarder to have a problem. "Each of us feels an emotional, and sometimes unhealthy, pull to the things we own," explains Robin Zasio, PsyD, LCSW, author of *The Hoarder in You*. "And we could all stand to be less attached to our possessions."

Easier said than done, though, because deep feelings are often behind those material objects. That old college sweatshirt you can't throw out represents more than just a cozy article of clothing, says Zasio. "It's part of your personal history, where you've been and who you are. Letting go can sometimes feel as though you're giving up a piece of yourself." Other possessions can represent achievement (say, a designer handbag collection that conveys a certain status) or security, especially in today's shaky economic climate.

But consumeristic tendencies can lead to both physical and emotional, well, baggage. "Having too many things can take up mental space and energy that you could be spending elsewhere," says Zasio. What's more, "studies have found that the more people are focused on possessions, the lower their personal well-being," says Tim Kasser, PhD, author of *The High Price of Materialism*. Not only are these people less satisfied with their lives, but they also have less energy and are more likely to smoke, use alcohol to excess, and suffer physical problems such as headaches and stomachaches.

Not a pretty picture, right? So if you want to lessen the power your possessions have over you, read on.

Step 1:
Recognize the Problem

Stuff overload doesn't happen overnight. It creeps up on us, like holiday pounds or credit-card debt. Some key signs of trouble:

You'll deal with it … later. Clutter can be a result of procrastination: Rather than handling things in the moment, we put them aside and save them for later. "A lot of us hang on to things because we imagine we'll use them one day, once we get them repaired or need them again," says Zasio. "But that never seems to happen." Assign an expiration date to each project on your to-do list, and if you haven't sewed that ripped skirt, or opened that book you meant to read, by your self-imposed deadline, return, donate, or toss the item in question.

You're consistently late or missing appointments. This can happen if you have too many clothes or accessories, which can make getting dressed a nightmare. "When there are too many choices, you spend too much time making decisions," says Dorothy Breininger, a member of and lecturer for the National Association of Professional Organizers and the Institute for Challenging Disorganization. Not only does it slow you down, but it's also mentally exhausting.

You have three unopened bottles of your favorite nail polish—and just bought more. If you don't have a real memory problem, you could be stockpiling. This behavior can be triggered by the thrill of a deal—such as buying it every time it goes on sale—or by an irrational fear that you might one day run out.

Step 2: Make Over Your Mind-Set

These tips can help get your coveting under control.

Focus on acquiring experiences, not things. Spending money on activities, such as a vacation or dinner out with friends, rather than material goods makes people happier in the long run, according to a study at San Francisco State University. "Think of it as investing in a happiness bank," says study author Ryan Howell, PhD, a quantitative psychologist at the university's Personality and Well-Being Lab. "You get the initial pleasure of doing something you enjoy, and then you can relive those feel-good moments again and again as memories." Objects, on the other hand, tend to lose their appeal over time because we get bored with them.

Remember this: Sometimes less really is more. Many people find comfort or familiarity in the quantity of their belongings rather than in the quality of them. It's the physical nature of the clutter—as opposed to what the clutter comprises—that can make it hard to let go. But the more you own, the less personal each object becomes and the easier it is to take it for granted. "Focus instead on investing in objects you really love and can't live without, instead of amassing things that have little meaning to you," says Breininger.

Get a purging partner. Have a friend or a neutral third party sit with you while you sift through the boxes. "Someone who is not so emotionally attached to the possessions can be more objective about figuring out what stays and what goes," says Breininger.

Step 3: Know What Needs to Go

Unless you're living in a monastery, odds are you have a few possessions that could stand being offloaded. Here's help in deciding what's expendable.

Do you use it often, or do you have something better that serves the same purpose? It might be a perfectly decent sweater, but if it's no longer in regular rotation, ditch it.

Exception: Is it for a special situation? Some items, like certain lingerie and lobster pots,

aren't suited for everyday use, but they have their time and place.

Is it sentimental? Memory-inducing items get a pass, as long as the memories are good ones and you can fit the stuff in two boxes. A pair of your baby shoes and your wedding album? Definite saves. Every airplane ticket from every trip you've ever been on? Chuck 'em.

Are you afraid to get rid of it? "Our brain chemistry is largely anxiety driven," says Zasio. "So we tend to think, *If I let this go, I may regret it.*" But if that's your only reason for keeping an item, it isn't reason enough.

Step 4: Clear the Clutter

Ready to begin tossing? Try these tricks for starters.

Don't handle things more than once. Every item you touch should either be put in its proper place or eliminated (read: recycled, donated, returned, or put into the trash). Don't decide to decide later.

Follow the "one in, one out" rule. Simply put, for each item you buy (say, a new pair of pumps), toss a corresponding item (that "so last season" pair).

Put a lid on it. Cap possessions by number (say, five pairs of jeans), size (one basketful of toiletries), or time (unread books will be donated after 3 months).

Clutter-Clearing Secrets from the Pros

Ready to excise the excess? Follow these organizing tips from the experts.

Stuff—we're all swimming in it, maybe even drowning in it: Stacks of paper seem to breed overnight. Opening a closet door means ducking an avalanche of clothes or towels from overstuffed shelves. And perhaps it's best not to discuss the Tupperware situation.

A home full of disarray and disorganization can consume your time, money, and energy. Fortunately, it doesn't have to be that way. Clutter expert and best-selling author Peter Walsh has been inside hundreds of homes in an effort to help people liberate themselves from the oppressive weight of "stuff." And purging all of those excess materials has resulted in all sorts of positive spin-off effects, he says. Many people report losing weight without even dieting, experiencing reenergized relationships, and even getting in better financial health. Want to finally lighten your load of stuff and find out how it can lighten and brighten your own life? Follow these tips from Walsh and other personal organizers.

Tackle the Worst Offenders

Most clutter falls into these four categories, according to Walsh—and he has a quick fix for each.

CLOTHES Walsh says a typical person wears 20% of their clothing 80% of the time. That means there's a whole lot of unused stuff cluttering your closet—one of the most stressful places in your home.

Quick Fix Try the reverse clothes hanger trick: Turn all of the clothes hanging in your closet so that the hangers face back-to-front. For the next 6 months, if you wear an item of clothing, return it to the closet with the hanger facing the correct way. "No cheating. If you try it on but decide not to wear it, make sure you put it back with the hanger turned backwards," Walsh advises.

After 6 months, look at which clothes are on hangers that are still facing in reverse—clothes you have not worn—and seriously consider getting rid of them all, Walsh says.

TOYS Anyone with children knows it can take only a matter of months for kid stuff to totally overrun the home. That doesn't have to be the norm, though. And decluttering won't just liberate Mom and Dad but will also help the kids feel better.

Quick Fix First, agree on a reasonable volume of toys. Set regular calendar reminders to sort through all toys and decide which will get passed on to another family or donated. Arrange the toys in distinct piles, either toy by toy, by age appropriateness, or by length of time the child has had the toy. Then team up with the kids to decide what should stay or go. Schedule a purge right before a birthday or the holidays, too, to clear away unused toys (and outgrown clothes) to make way for a few new items.

KITCHEN GADGETS It's time to rethink the pickle picker, plastic butter-spreading contraptions,

and countless corncob holders. You may even need to part with that treasured quesadilla maker.

Quick Fix Take Walsh's 1-Month Cardboard Box Test: Empty the contents of your utensil drawers into a cardboard box. For 1 month, return a utensil to the drawer only if you take it out of the box to use it. At the end of the month, seriously consider discarding everything that's still in the box. "Face it—if it's still in the box after 4 weeks, you don't need it," Walsh says. "Pass it on

Get Hooked

Hooks such as 3M Command adhesives can help you take and keep control of your closet. They keep hangables off the floor and help you see more of your accessories and bags. Use them solo or make them multipurpose with these tips.

Hook + Sturdy Hanger: Place a hanger on the hook, then drape scarves or belts side by side on it. They'll all be visible at once instead of hidden in a pile.

Hook + Plastic Rings: Link a set of shower-curtain rings, then hang the top one from a hook. Slide drapables (like tees) through each to maximize vertical space.

Hook + Mini Pouch: Store shirt buttons, shoe inserts, or little extras in a small bag hung on a hook so you know where to find them immediately.

to charity." (One exception: the turkey baster. Hold on to that one—you'll need it in November!)

THE GARAGE "Clutter is decisions delayed." That's one of Walsh's favorite sayings. And nowhere is this more apparent than the garage, which is often used for long-term storage of stuff we think we want but don't know what to do with: broken gadgets waiting for repair, magazines we swear we'll one day read, and possessions handed down from loved ones.

Quick Fix Do Walsh's Trash Bag Tango: Grab two trash bags and set a timer for 10 minutes. Fill one bag with recyclables or things that need to go in the trash, like broken toys. Fill the other with items to donate. If you and another person do that daily for a week, you'll end up with 14 bags of trash/recyclables and 14 bags of donations.

Another key step: labeling. Since the garage is often used for stashing seasonal items, sports equipment, and holiday decorations, be sure to clearly label boxes and containers. Walsh suggests color coding, too, such as orange for Halloween decorations and white for holiday lights.

Finally, for clutter you believe holds nostalgic, emotional, or sentimental value, pick two or three treasures that remind you of a particular person or memory—that give you joy and pleasure—and donate the rest. "Bring them out of the dark and frame or display them in a way that treats them with honor or respect," Walsh suggests. "You'll be amazed at how it takes the power out of the rest of the stuff."

The Reject Pile

Once it's a no, where should it go?
- **Good stuff you're just over:** Clothes-swap party! "Get together with friends around your size for this," suggests professional organizer Amy Trager.
- **Worn-once cocktail dress:** Bring it to a secondhand store. If it's in great condition, fashionable, and in season, you could get about 15% of the retail price when it sells.
- **Your first power suit:** Donate it to Dress for Success, a nonprofit that helps disadvantaged women suit up for, then ace, job interviews. DFS affiliates are nearly nationwide, but if there isn't one where you live, research local equivalents.

Practice What Pros Preach

These tricks of the trade can help you transform a cluttered space into an organized area—and keep the chaos from creeping back.

TAKE STOCK OF YOUR STORAGE Some home organizers recommend never buying any storage items and, instead, simply getting rid of anything that needs storing. Beth Carmichael, a designer and organizer whose business, Three Horseshoes, is based in Sydney, Nova Scotia, doesn't go to that extreme: "It's unrealistic that a person wouldn't want to save some things. But you probably have all of the storage containers and shelving you need—you just need to clear out what you have."

INVENTORY YOUR WASTE Do you find yourself consistently throwing away half of the deli meat you buy or overbrowned bananas from your fruit bowl? "Careful purchasing is key to living an organized life," says Candace Greer, a personal organizer and owner of Art and Order in Lafayette, LA. She recommends keeping an inventory of perishables that you throw away to help you get control of your grocery shopping and your pantry.

Follow the same rule while you clear out bureaus and bathroom cabinets: Do you find yourself buying, but not wearing, workout gear or tank tops? Do you purchase far more hand lotion and makeup than you use? Keep track to save yourself both money and time.

KNOW YOUR LIMITS Greer does a lot of closet excavation projects and often finds that clients have a favorite go-to look, which they tend to buy in multiples. "They may not even realize they have this many until we clear them out," she says. But she encourages clients to slim it down to just three of each. Beyond that, it's truly just clutter. Ask yourself: Do you really need more than three white button-down shirts?

PLAN A PRE-EVENT PURGE Spring cleaning is great, says organizer Renée Ory, of Amazing Spaces in Lafayette, LA, but it makes even more sense to coordinate sprucing up with events—everything from cleaning out your refrigerator before you grocery shop (remember to inventory that waste!) to sorting through toys ahead of birthdays and winter holidays. Before shopping for back-to-school clothes, empty out your child's dresser and discard or donate clothes that are hopelessly ripped or stained or no longer fit.

BE REALISTIC ABOUT EBAY That box full of items you've been saving ... and saving ... because you're sure you could sell them on

Craigslist or eBay? The experts' consensus: Donate them. "You've had this box for how long?" asks Carmichael. "Yeah, you're not going to sell it." That can be hard to accept, so Greer suggests setting a time limit: "If they're not up there and listed in 2 weeks, Goodwill gets them."

DIVIDE AND CONQUER "Never pull everything out of your closet at once," says Jamie Novak, author of *1,000 Best Quick and Easy Organizing Secrets*. You'll run out of time, motivation, or both. Instead, set a timer for 15 to 20 minutes and try to get through just one section, like your jeans or your jewelry, in a single sitting.

SHARE THE JOY In her best-selling book, *The Life-Changing Magic of Tidying Up*, Marie Kondo tackles clutter and tangled emotions with a simple edict: If an item does not bring you joy, let it go—and let go of any ensuing guilt, too. "If someone gave you a gift, and you opened it and felt joy at that moment, that can be enough," says Carmichael. "Plus, passing on the gift brings another person joy," she says. Keeping gifts that have limited use for you, whether they don't fit or just don't work in your life, is not necessary and can cause lingering guilt.

NIX IT, DON'T BOX IT Ory recommends finding cute ways to display favorite objects: shadowboxes for precious baby items, clustered vacation souvenirs mounted on the wall. But she says that once things get placed in a box and covered with a lid, they could better be donated: You don't need them. Carmichael is similarly minimalistic, recommending a single box of keepsakes per child—just some heirloom objects and a few particularly special art projects per school year. No one needs every aced spelling test or every drawing by a prolific sketcher.

KEEP IT SIMPLE In their early attempts at home organization, many people try to incorporate systems that are too complex to keep up, particularly with filing systems for bills. "They come up with these methods that end up with one piece of paper per folder," says Greer. "For any kind of organization system, I go with the KISS rule: Keep It Simple, Silly. If it's too complicated, it falls apart fast."

It's equally crucial to follow an easy plan for clearing items out. Organizational methods sometimes list as many as seven categories for items, but Carmichael vehemently opposes that approach: "Three piles is the best way: keep, donate, discard. Any system more complicated than this simply gets too difficult. It won't work."

GO FOR QUALITY, NOT QUANTITY

When Greer goes on vacation, she seeks out a single higher-end piece of local art instead of a half-dozen ornaments, tchotchkes, and T-shirts. "It's a more meaningful souvenir that's easier to display than a million tiny things. And when it all adds up, the piece of art can even be cheaper."

This philosophy applies to your closet, too: It's always better to buy one well-made pair of shoes than several cheap, trendy styles that probably hurt your feet anyway. "The same absolutely goes for handbags and clothes," says Greer.

FOCUS ON FUNCTION, NOT TRADITION

Ory coaches clients to think realistically about the way their lives function and how to work within the space they have. Some clients, for example, prefer to get dressed in the bathroom after their morning shower. In that case, it makes sense to keep underwear in the bathroom, if space allows, rather than the bedroom. "Think functional and think in zones," she says. There's no reason to follow rules that don't make sense for your lifestyle.

AIM FOR PROGRESS, NOT PERFECTION

Though some organizational methods—most notably Kondo's—encourage a massive onetime cleanout, Greer encourages a more realistic, incremental outlook. "Just give yourself a project, a goal, and a timeline—say, 30 minutes and a bookshelf," she advises. "You're going for progress, not perfection, and as you do more, you'll be inspired to keep going."

FEEL RELIEF, NOT REGRET

"You do not need to keep every object with sentimental value," says Ory. If you're feeling heartless and worried about forgetting the memories associated with an object, she recommends taking a picture. Losing items means gaining space, a worthy tradeoff. "Space in your home gives you a sense of peace that no object can give you," says Carmichael.

"Never once have I had a client come back and tell me that they regret getting rid of something," says Greer. "Not once."

7 Days, 7 Ways to a **Serene Space**

A plan to create order from chaos in just 1 week

No idea where to begin? This weeklong program prescribes a doable daily dose of clutter control. If 7 days in a row is simply too much, too soon, take 7 Saturdays in a row. Just stick with it—finally kicking a clutter habit will be well worth the effort.

Monday: Organize Your Inbox

Slip into the office an hour early for an uninterrupted cleaning session. Activate your out-of-office email reply and turn off the auto chime for 2 hours. Create new electronic folders for contacts, projects, and meetings. Sort alphabetically, then redirect emails to folders or delete them (after all, 80% of work email is unnecessary). In the future, be relentless and begin filing/deleting emails on arrival. When you get a request for a project update, the information will be only a click away.

Tuesday: Calm Cabinet Chaos

Roll up your sleeves and tackle your kitchen cabinets. Gather two cardboard boxes. Place punch bowls and platters you haven't used in months in basement- or yard sale–bound boxes. Replace cabinet linings and sift through cans, teas, and cracker boxes, throwing out the expired and moving older cans to the front. Pour flour, cereal, and sugar into transparent plastic containers to keep them fresh and protected against bugs.

Wednesday:
Create a Hassle-Free Hall Closet

Plow through the gear crowding the hall closet. Pair up miscellaneous shoes and place them on a door hanger; chuck sports equipment into large wicker baskets and move them to the garage; discard worn-out sneakers. Group similar items such as umbrellas in a round container. And keep it seasonal: If sweltering temps have you in tank tops every day, relegate the winter woollies to plastic storage boxes.

Thursday: Conquer the Linen Closet

Pull out all like items and organize your linens by shelf. Keep towels together and group by type: washcloths, hand towels, bath towels, etc. If tattered towels are in the mix, tear them into cleaning rags. Keep top sheets separate from bottom sheets. Put any appliances—hair dryers, irons, curlers—on another shelf and toiletries on yet another.

Friday: Manage Your Meds

Sort through the prescriptions in your medicine cabinet. Trash expired drugs and throw out lotions and cosmetics you haven't used in the past 3 months or so. Put cotton swabs and cotton balls in easy-to-reach glass containers. Replace hand soaps and toothbrushes; stock extras for unexpected houseguests.

Saturday: Draft Your Family

Time to extend your organization to the family. Outline a cleaning schedule with weekly and monthly tasks for each person. Create incentives: Pitch in and clean today, hit the amusement park next Saturday. Give each family member a job: vacuum, dust, do the laundry, get rid of outdated newspapers. Finish at noon and switch to relaxation mode.

Sunday: Plot Your Pleasures

This day is all about you! Order takeout, play your favorite tunes, and resist the boob tube. In a notebook, scribble wish lists: books and magazines to read, movies to see, restaurants to try, old friends to call. Think about the people and places you want to visit in the coming year (keeping in mind what's realistic and affordable). Then grab your calendar and schedule your trips.

Pare Down, Drop Pounds

A cluttered kitchen could sabotage weight loss—how to clean up and slim down.

Your kitchen isn't the enemy in your quest for healthy weight loss. It's the clutter in your kitchen that's the problem. Case in point: In an *Environment and Behavior* study, when women hung out in messy kitchens, they mindlessly snacked on twice as much junk food as those who were in tidy ones. (Chew on that for a moment.) These eight tips for organizing your kitchen will help you cut calories without even thinking about it.

I. DON'T KEEP CEREAL ON TOP OF THE FRIDGE The top of the refrigerator seems like the most convenient spot for those oversize boxes, right? But even if they don't come plastered with rainbows, horseshoes, clovers, and balloons, storing them out in the open could mean serious weight gain. Women who store cereal where they can see it are 21 pounds heavier, on average, than those who keep it more or less hidden away in cabinets or pantries, says Brian Wansink, PhD, director of the Cornell Food and Brand Lab and author of *Slim by Design*. That's because simply seeing food can trigger people to eat it, says clinical psychologist Susan Albers, author of *50 More Ways to Soothe Yourself Without Food*.

2. GET THE TV OUT OF THERE Beyond taking up valuable real estate in your kitchen, TVs distract you into overeating, says Georgie Fear, RD, author of *Lean Habits for Lifelong Weight Loss*. Your brain doesn't recognize how much food you're eating or let you know when you're full, which is a one-two punch to your weight loss goals. Distracted eating even puts you at risk of overeating at subsequent meals, according to research published in the Journal of Health Psychology. After all, if your brain didn't register everything you ate at dinner, it's more apt to crave a midnight snack.

3. IGNORE THE CRISPER DRAWER "Promote the fruit and vegetables in your fridge by getting them up to eye level," says Fear. "Give that zucchini and kale a starring role at center stage." You're nearly three times more likely to eat healthy foods if they're in your line of sight, says Wansink. Your produce might not last quite as long outside the crisper, but chances are you'll end up throwing out less slimy spinach.

4. BE TRANSPARENT ABOUT YOUR FRUIT While you're emptying out that fruit drawer, place any easy-to-snack-on produce that holds up well at room temperature (like apples, bananas, oranges, and mangoes) in a clear fruit bowl, says Albers. In one *Health Education and Behavior* study, women who kept fresh fruit on the counter weighed 13 pounds less than those whose kitchens were fruit bowl–free. Just make sure it's in a highly visible spot, not tucked in the corner with your stand mixer.

5. FILL UP YOUR FREEZER Let's be honest: Sometimes you open the refrigerator meaning to grab a Greek yogurt and somehow end up holding a pan of left-over cheesecake. Try keeping less-than-nourishing foods in the freezer—since you tend to hit that less frequently—to reduce those derailed trips to the fridge, says Fear. Or limit your in-fridge storage to a single serving, she says—automatic portion control.

6. NIX THE KNICKKNACKS A collection of puppy figurines can be ridiculously cute. But anything that clutters your kitchen—even if it's not edible—can increase your chances of emotional eating. That's because, according to Wansink's study, your brain registers clutter as chaos, and that leads to a major increase in food intake. Embrace minimalist decor.

7. HIDE CONTAINERS' CONTENTS Not everyone is lucky enough to have a Pinterest-worthy kitchen with huge cabinets and a walk-in pantry. "If you must have containers on your counters, use ceramic jars," Albers says. "They are stackable, meaning they take up less counter space, and you cannot see through them." In one *Obesity* study, women ate half as many chocolates when they were stored in opaque versus see-through containers.

INSIDE:
Your Live Well, Die Happy Guides

Live every day of your life to the fullest!

GUIDE I
Drug-Free Fixes: Natural Solutions for Pain Relief

Turn to kitchen cures to banish annoying aches and pains without drug-induced side effects, and use soothing moves and gentle self-massage to help knock out pain—fast!

GUIDE 2
Think Yourself Happy & Healthy

Get grounded, discover true joy, and bolster your health with a simple, time-proven technique. Discover nature's best therapies for boosting mood and slashing stress. Make the most of every single day by following the hour-by-hour guide.

GUIDE 3
Clear Out the Clutter

Longing to get organized? Follow these secrets from the pros, including seven ways to create a serene space in just a week. Bonus: Learn how whittling down your possessions can help you slim down, too.

Find all that—and more!—in these three guides!

202966601
LiveWellDieHappy/AR/4-17
Printed in USA

001921